Dedication

This book is dedicated to my father, Earl Hampton. He died of lung cancer in 1993. I really miss him. He always said, "If you do something; do it right, or just don't do it at all".

Love to my husband, Keevin; to my sounding board, my mother, Hilda Hampton. To my children, Keevin, Kimisha and Kenton. (Thanks Kimisha for your special encouragement.)

And special thanks to my staff at Davis Medical Group, Inc.; my patients and all who inspired me.

Most of all, love to God for His everlasting guidance and direction.

ACKNOWLEDGEMENTS

Once again, I want to thank the staff at Davis Medical Group, Inc. for their encouragement and support.

Special thanks:

-to Valerie Brown. I want to thank you for your special insight and skill that helped me complete this book. Your enthusiasm with the revisions was incredible.

-to Deborah Wise and Barbara Butler. Thank you for being my sounding boards. You really helped to keep me focused.

-to Melita Ellis. You kept saying, "Dr. Davis, you've got to write the book." Well, I wrote the book! Thank you. Your spiritual support was appreciated.

-to Marie Love. Thank you for nurturing not only me but my patients as well.

-to Lenore Cunningham. Your quiet and serene calmness has provided just the right balance for me. Thank you.

-to Jean Moses. The energy and enthusiasm that you have shared daily as you have succeeded in your restoration has been phenomenal. You have truly been an inspiration to me and hundreds of others.

-to Dr. Carolyn Mazloomi. Your insight has been invaluable.

-to Kathleen Gallon. Your insight and intuitiveness was so greatly needed and appreciated.

-Holly Sowels. Your passion for perfection makes you a wonderful editor. Out of our association; a new friendship has developed, for that I am grateful.

TABLE OF CONTENTS

Note from the author........................... 9

Important Information.......................... 11

Introduction.....................................13

Chapter 1
Why Are We So Sick?........................ 17

Chapter 2
Food That Make Us Sick....................... 27

Chapter 3
So What's Left? What Can We Eat?...... 43

Chapter 4
Exercise At Its Best............................ 61

Chapter 5
Get Out Of The Shower......................... 67

Chapter 6
Let's Put It All Together......................... 73

Chapter 7
Vitamins and Minerals............................ 79

Chapter 8
Anoint Thyself With Oils......................... 87

Chapter 9
Conditions and Diseases and Remedies..95

Chapter 10
Guidelines For Good Health...................109

Testimonials..143

Quick Tips... 151

Reference Guide...................................... 169

Note From The Author

Today, at age 43, I am as vibrant, youthful and energetic as I was seventeen years ago on my wedding day.

Being a physician, I know that good health is no accident. A few years ago, after taking inventory of my own body condition and health status, I began research into health, wellness and restoration. I took the best of all I learned and incorporated the easiest and fastest methods into my lifestyle. Let's face it, if it's not fast and easy, we're not going to stick with anything. I lost weight while improving my overall health.

As many of my patients were having the same experience, I developed a program that they could follow, see and feel results and maintain those results. This is not just about weight loss. It's about good health and body restoration. It's like finding a fountain of youth.

Certain conditions and diseases can be prevented or reversed. The skin will be restored to it's optimal condition; smooth as a 'baby's bottom'.

I have outlined everything in an easy to follow format that will allow you to experience what I, as well as my patients, have discovered. Take time to read the testimonials even before you read the book. They alone will motivate you to start your own journey to good *health, wellness and restoration.*

IMPORTANT INFORMATION

The information and recommendations in this book do not apply to everyone. The genetic makeup of particular individuals may predispose them to certain reactions. Discontinue this program if you develop any adverse reactions.

Do not self-diagnose or self-medicate without the specific guidance of a physician and/or a qualified herbalist.

The author, publisher and distributors will not be held responsible for any adverse side effects, reactions, consequences or claims that evolve from the use of the suggestions or recommendations contained in this book.

Obtain a complete physical examination from your doctor; including blood work to analyze your blood sugar, cholesterol level, thyroid level, blood type and special blood chemistries. This is important so that your physician may check for any underlying diseases and to give you a starting point for your restoration program.

I highly recommend that you read "Eat Right For Your Type" by Dr. Peter J. D'Adamo in conjunction with this book for optimal results. Dr. D'Adamo's book is the most up-to-date information source that explains how foods, beverages and exercises effects your health according to your specific blood type.

After reading this book you will be ready to get started on the program. There are several items that I suggest you secure before you begin:

Natural bristle brush; Peppermint soap; Ezekiel 4:9 bread (available at health food stores)
Books for reference:
Dr. Atkin's New Revolutionary Diet - Dr. Robert Atkins
Fitonics For Life by Marilyn Diamond
Eat Right 4 Your Type-Dr. Peter J. D'Adamo
Prescriptions For Nutritional Healing - Dr. James Balch

Keep all medicine, oils and herbs from the reach of children. Consult a physician before placing children on this program.

INTRODUCTION

I've always prayed that God would allow me to be an instrument that would help people all over the world. Never did I expect Him to entrust me with something so important, something so special. It's what we've all been looking for - restoration, good health, inner peace and spiritual happiness.

I wrote this book so that people, all people, from all walks of life, can understand and improve the quality of their lives, their parents' lives, their children's lives and the lives of future generations.

I've always been interested in and fascinated with marketing. It has been to the point where I would wake up in the middle of the night and get these ideas of how a particular advertisement would work better. I always dwelled on getting their message; why did they use this symbol or color or even why was it arranged in the manner that it was. I finally realized why I was so interested and intrigued.

Our major health problems and conditions are so intimately related to the marketing industry and is the major economical-driving force in this country. As sad as it sounds, this country's advertising medium is instrumental in keeping us obese, fatigued, depressed, suicidal and hypertensive. They contribute to us having Attention Deficit Disorder, diabetes, irritable bowel, Alzheimer's, arthritis, gastritis, cancer, gout, fibromyalgia, chronic fatigue syndrome, heart disease, heart failure, strokes, renal failure and the list goes on.

The foods that are so heavily marketed are the same agents that are destroying our lives, our family's lives and the lives of future generations. You must realize that our country is a consuming country and we the people are the gross national product. We are the major factor that drives our economy. The cascade is a mighty element that keeps us economically strong.

Just look at the aggressive growth of the pharmaceutical industry alone in the last decade - record profits. Look at the sale of soda. Again, record profits. Before you complete this book you will understand why we are so sick and you'll know how we can undo the damage and live longer, healthier, more productive lives and assure the same healthy standard for the next generation.

This book is like no other you will encounter. It combines a program of reducing complex carbohydrates while increasing fruits, vegetables and fiber in the diet. It increases the use of herbs, oils and vitamins. It will employ skin conditioning and specific exercises. The program stimulates and improves the immune system, helps reduce excess weight, reduces the risk of certain diseases and in some cases has eliminated them altogether. It also helps increase physical and mental stamina.

I've made it very simple. I have hundreds of patients, their family members and friends across the country on this program and I'll share a few of their many successes. I will explain how the marketing industry drives our spending and eating habits. Once you see how everything fits, you'll be able to make the necessary adjustments.

CHAPTER 1

Why Are We So Sick?

"We are sick because of the foods we eat as well as the foods we fail to eat; the exercises we do and the exercises that we don't do."

Denise Davis, M.D.

There are certain foods and beverages that we eat every day that contribute to poor health and illness. The foods that I'm referring to are the complex carbohydrates. They are also known as complex sugars.

This list includes:

potatoes (white and red)
rice (white)
corn
breads
bananas
beets
carrots
pasta
cereal
coffee
soda
sugar
flour

These complex carbohydrates, once ingested, trigger the increase of the insulin in the blood. Insulin, a hormone excreted from the pancreas that regulates the metabolism of glucose and other nutrients, is necessary because it helps keep hormonal balance in the body. These foods; however, in the presentation and quantity that we ingest them in the good ole American diet, is literally killing us. We have diseases now in record numbers - diabetes, heart disease, allergies, strokes, cancer, obesity among adults and children. Our children are 60% overweight and their incidence of hypertension, cholesterol elevation, attention deficit and depression is at an all time high. Our children don't run or play actively. Children in other countries easily master three or four languages while ours barely master one. This is because of sluggish minds brought about by poor diet and lack of exercise. This is the result of three generations of fast food.

The insulin level increases once these foods are eaten. Prolonged increase in insulin does many things; many destructive things to our bodies.

Let's talk about Insulin:

* Insulin modifies and/or destroys receptors, therefore they do not respond to a sugar load effectively. These people become diabetics. Their sugar levels remain high. They must bring it down with diet, oral medication or insulin injections.

* Insulin can make the kidneys retain water and salt. These people can become hypertensive, bloated, fatigued or depressed. They complain of joint pain, migraine headaches, insomnia, arthritis, irritable bowel syndrome, Crohn's disease, memory loss, swelling of the hands and feet and a host of other complaints that come from fluid retention. Aging is accelerated by the retention of salt and water.

* Insulin can cause the migration of fat from these food in particular to go to storage in the fat cells. That accounts for

the overweight and obesity problems as well as aging.

* Insulin cause the fat from these foods to stay in the blood. This causes chronic fatigue, depression, high cholesterol and heart disease.

* Insulin makes the inner cells of the blood vessels swell. This causes the inner lumen of the vessel to thicken and swell. So the heart is pumping and working harder and harder to push the blood through this swollen vessel. This causes hypertension, migraine headaches, irritable bowel and any pain that throbs.

* Insulin can cause the increase in the release of a nerve hormone called neuroepinephrine, which innervates or controls the arteries. An increase in this hormone will make the arteries spasm and throb. This accounts for migraine headaches, fatigue, gastritis, irritable bowel syndrome, chest pain and gallbladder attacks.

* Insulin causes cells in various parts of the body to multiply and proliferate wildly. This accounts for fibroid tumors, arthritis, gastritis, fibromyalgia, multiple sclerosis, gallbladder disease, appendicitis, acne, endrometriosis and cancer.

I know that this is not a pretty picture but it is one you must look at. The portions and types of complex carbohydrates that we are consuming are escalating our diseased condition. Look at hypertension alone. We have poor vessels that are loaded with extra water, extra salt, extra fat. The heart is trying to pump the blood through vessels that are thickened on the inside and that are spasming. Now can you see why some people with hypertension often take several different types of medication?

So, at this point, we've identified for the first time how and where we get diseases. Depending on your particular genetic makeup (your unique makeup passed down to you by your parents and preceding generations) there are certain triggers which eventually give you one particular medical condition versus another. Foods definitely affect us. Environmental factors, such as the air, water, smog and smoke, can affect us also. Another factor that has a tremendous effect on us is stress.

STRESS

Stress is one factor that also can elevate the insulin level. Be it physical stress such as an injury or medical illness or mental stress such as depression, fatigue or anxiety, the insulin level elevates as a response. Therefore, stress will directly cause and magnify the whole cascade of diseases and illnesses that affect us everyday.

Case in point: Have you ever had a headache, stomach or joint pain after an argument or disagreement or at a time of personal stress or perhaps after a traumatic experience? If so, this is what happens: Physiologically, your insulin rises, the salt water make the brain tissue swell, the joints swell, the intestinal tissues swell, the vessels thicken and the vessels also pulsate.

Then, as a result, here comes the throbbing headache, the nausea, the gastritis, the cramping and the joint pain. See, it's all related. Once we learn to overcome stress, the trigger, the cascade diminishes. It's just that simple.

The beauty of this restorative program is that stress will decrease naturally as you follow the steps outlined.

CHAPTER 2

Foods That Make Us Sick

Bread and Pasta

"I love bread!   I love pasta!" Well, bread and pasta love you too.   These foods are tasty and are the base of our food pyramid. We are advised to eat 6 - 8 servings a day. Unfortunately, the portions and the time of day we eat these foods are detrimental to our health. The chemical used to bleach the flour (chlorine) can cause allergies, hypertension, hair loss and a host of other problems.

Bread and pasta are approximately ten thousand years old and the human race is older than that.   These are not foods that grow naturally so perhaps we should approach them with extreme caution.   It takes work to process these foods so they can be eaten. Our creator did not intend for it to be so difficult.

Potatoes, Carrots & Beets

Potatoes are the   mainstay of most people's diets. They grow underground as do carrots and beets.   These complex carbohydrates break down to pure sugar that increases the blood insulin level. So perhaps we should not eat them in the quantities that they are consumed. They should only be eaten at the evening meal; for that lessens the insulin effect.

Rice

Rice (white) involves an eleven step elaborate process to come to our plates. It is not easily obtained and it elevates blood insulin levels.

A common question arises concerning people who consume large quantities of rice and still appear to be in good health. Although rice itself may create higher insulin levels; the gravy, butter, salt or other condiments that Americans add to rice only serve to worsen this condition. Another point to be stressed is that Americans usually eat meat along with their rice. The size steak that the average U.S. consumer eats at a restaurant would be enough to feed a family of five for several meals in other countries. That is because they use the meat as a condiment to flavor or season, not as the primary food. Many countries view eating large quantities of food as gluttonous and distasteful. Got the picture? Combining meat with a complex carbohydrate actually slows down the metabolism and contributes to weight gain and fatigue.

Corn

Years ago, corn had small kernels and was not necessarily sweet. Now, corn is genetically altered such that it results in large kernels that are extremely sweet due to its high sugar content. High sugar means high insulin reaction.

What About Cereal?

Yes, let's talk about cereal. Processed cereal - you know the brands. My question to you is: Was cereal around when man first inhabited the earth? No. It wasn't here. Corn cereal was discovered by accident about one hundred years ago. Now, hundreds of brands line our grocery shelves and in some stores, down both aisles. Processed cereal is a new food which drives the insulin level up.

Saturday mornings, the cartoon stations blast our children with commercials pushing the cereals, most of which are loaded with sugar. No wonder children suffer from Attention Deficit Disorder. Some parents fill their children with cereal coupled with toast and bananas. No wonder they are so sluggish around one to three o'clock in the afternoon. Do you remember how you felt at fifth period after lunch? It was hard for teachers as well as students to stay awake.

Cereal, like the other complex carbohydrates listed, slows the metabolism down and increases the insulin level. Their content comes from the corn, wheat or rice, as well as the sugar which may coat certain brands. It has an additive effect.

What About Bananas?

I'm going to tell you a lot of things about bananas. Some of them may surprise you and you may find them hard to believe.

Bananas, I found through much research, are one of, if not the most lethal foods one can eat. Let's really talk about the banana.

Bananas are fruits native to tropical areas, such as parts of Africa and South America in deep forests and jungles. They have a bitter tasting thin membrane or string you pull off the banana. Well, that bitter taste comes from a chemical that can irritate the gums. Depending on the acid content of your saliva, that chemical may also leach the enamel of your teeth.

Bananas are definitely part of the marketing strategy of our grocery stores. They are usually in as many as six locations within the store. While all other fruits have one location. You'll find them where you first get your cart, the produce section, the check out lane; the dairy section, the meat section and finally in the cereal aisle. They are on sale in most stores for nineteen cents a pound each week. Bananas stay on sale because they bring consumers to the grocery store as often as twice a week. Have you noticed that they do not stay fresh as long as they use to? It seems as if I remember them lasting about a week compared to the three to fours day they last now. So when people come back to the store for more, they also pick up other items while they are at the store. Smart marketing.

Adults love bananas. They are quick and simple. You don't have to clean a banana or use a knife to cut it. It is self contained. No other fruit has the shape of a banana. It's oblong while other fruits are round or oval. Oranges are round, apples are round, grapes are round, watermelons are round, melons are round - bananas have an odd shape. The banana is the only fresh fruit that does not make juice when eaten. All other fruits make juice.

With its odd shape and unique properties, it seems to me that bananas are more suited for consumption by our relatives, the monkeys. As monkeys live high in trees and travel from branch to branch, the banana can be easily grabbed and held onto. The banana's sickle shape enables the monkey to pass it to other relatives high in the trees; thus having food and nourishment without having to come down among its predators. If the banana was juicy, the monkey would constantly urinate on its relatives on the lower branches. And on the other hand, the fact that the banana causes constipation, prevents the monkey from defecating on those lower branch relatives. Need I say more?

You may ask, what about potassium?

Yes, what about your potassium? For years doctors have instructed patients to eat one or two bananas a day for the potassium. Let me tell you a much better source of potassium. It's a little fruit called kiwi.

Kiwis have more potassium than the banana. The banana has 400 milligrams of potassium; the kiwi has 480 milligrams. Kiwi has more vitamin C than an orange. The banana can cause constipation and fatigue; the kiwi will keep you regular because it has more fiber than seven bowls of oatmeal. The banana will keep weight on you because of the greater number of calories; the kiwi aids weight loss with its less number of calories. The kiwi is also higher in fiber content. The banana significantly effects the insulin level elevation. It raises the insulin level and keeps it up longer than any of the foods listed.

Any food that keeps poisons and toxins in the body for long periods of time contributes to heart disease, hypertension, high cholesterol, weight gain and cancer (our major diseases).

What's wrong with soda?

Soda has no nutritional value. Again, it is a man-made, processed product that was not medically designed for our bodies. It contains about twelve teaspoons of sugar, artificial color and artificial flavors. Soda has nothing to nourish your cells to protect you against depression, diabetes, hypertension or cancer. It has no value. Diet soda has no carbohydrates with its artificial sweeteners. It is also made of phosphoric acid, carbon dioxide and methane gas! This is the carbonation that puts the "kick" in the soda. Diet soda increases the appetite. Phosphoric acid leaches the calcium from the bones and is responsible for the increase in the record number of cases of gallstones, kidney stones, bone fractures and most recently, osteoporosis.

Let's examine the marketing of soda. Years ago if a customer wanted more soda after the initial purchase in a restaurant, they would have to pay full price for another one. Now, once the initial purchase is made, the customer can get an unlimited amount of free refills. Ever fill the cup and walk out of the restaurant with a fresh cup of soda? Why is that? Rent has gone up, food has gone up, taxes have gone up; why is soda free? Well, when people drink soda, it increases their appetite; they eat more food, buy more often and buy bigger quantities. This has given birth to the super-sized or big value meals. It all ties to money. Again, the more soda that we consume, the more the insulin cascade is activated, Therefore, the medical problems increase and that spurs the economy. Again, it all ties to money.

Soda is sold in an average of seven locations in the store:

1. Outside the building are life-size machines of soda (4 to 6 machines minimum).

2. Cart area - 24-can displays when you first walk into the store.

3. Soda aisle - displayed on both sides.

4. Cereal aisle - Let's face it, children tell us what to buy.

5. Deli area - get a quick sandwich to go and grab a soda.

6. Salad bar - quick salads and pick up a soda.

7. Checkout lane - Grab a soda to drink as you checkout your groceries and also to drink while you drive home.

Soda - always on sale, super-sized cups in convenient stores and usually the only beverage up until recently offered at the movies. There are more cans and bottles of soda sold than individual eggs. That's amazing and very sad.

Soda for breakfast, soda for lunch, soda for snack, soda with dinner, soda before bedtime. Let's face it; every since there has been a proliferation of bagel shops, coffee shops, free refills and super-sized portions, American people have literally blown up; not only in size but also with diseases.

Sugar

Studies show that the average American adult consumes an average of 150 pounds of sugar per year. Teens are known to consume twice that amount. Does that surprise you? Sugar is hidden in about every convenience food that we consume. Low-fat foods often mean higher sugar. Read the labels. Refined sugar, whether in the "pure" form or altered form (powdered or brown) leads to many of our health problems. Sugar, when ingested, directly increases blood insulin levels and the cascade that follows, including obesity, diabetes, hypertension, depression, heart disease, tooth decay, constipation, arthritis, fibromyalgia, insomnia, hyperactivity, infections, varicose veins, aging, migraine headaches, allergies, pre-eclampsia, and the list goes on and on.

Artificial sweeteners are free from carbohydrates and calories. They don't elevate the blood insulin like sugar; however, aspartame, a chemical in these sweeteners, virtually increases the appetite and increases thirst especially when sodas are ingested. Methanol, an alcohol, a key component in aspartame, can cause depression, headaches, irritability, blurred vision, tachycardia, nausea, insomnia, gastritis, edema and numbness of the extremities and joints. Do any of these symptoms sound familiar? Studies have suggested an association of blindness with this chemical. So choose sweeteners with caution. We should use more unrefined sweeteners such as date sugar, rice sugar, cane sugar and honey. And don't be afraid to eat foods with no sweetener. You may be surprised to find that many foods are quite tasty in their natural form!

CHAPTER 3

So What's Left?
What Can We Eat?

Breakfast

Let's all go back to bed and figure this out. At night our body is healing and repairing itself. In the morning some wonderful things happen as the result of what the body has been doing while we've slept. We have crystals in our eyes, wax in our ears, mucus in our nose, crystals in our nose, a film on our teeth, our breath stinks, we urinate, defecate, pass gas - sounds very graphic but yes, we get the stuff out, right? Well, the first thing our bodies want and need is something sweet, wet, clean and refreshing, a piece of fruit. Anything but a banana of course. A piece of fruit that will clean, deodorize, energize and rejuvenate the intestinal tract before we become active for the day.

The best fruits that burn fat are listed below:

-melon
-kiwi
-strawberries
-blueberries

-blackberries
-boysenberries
-raspberries
-plums
-pineapples
-lemons
-grapefruit
-papaya

Apples, oranges, grapes, mangoes, etc. are excellent fruits. However, they do not burn fat like the ones listed above.

The other thing the body needs in the morning is protein. The proteins are the energy foods. The fats of the protein sources are necessary fats that line the nerves, lubricate the organs, keeps your skin soft and keeps your hair from falling out. Poor thyroid function can store fats due to an extremely slow metabolic rate. These fats within a person with a normal metabolic rate do not increase the insulin; therefore, they do not get stored.

Here you may wish to refer to Dr. D'Adamo's book ("Eat Right For Your

Type") so you can make the wisest choices for your meals according to your specific blood type.

Protein list:

- meat: beef, pork, fish, poultry
- soy products
- cheese
- eggs
- nuts
- cottage cheese
- yogurt

So an ideal breakfast would incorporate choices from these groups. Vegetable are also good breakfast food choices. They are loaded with nutrients and low in carbohydrates, calories and fat. Leftover veggies from last night's dinner make quick and healthy breakfasts. Use your imagination.

Don't Limit Yourself

Fish and chicken, especially fish, suppresses the appetite more than any other food choice. When you select these protein foods as breakfast, they naturally suppress the appetite for the day as well as giving energy to the body to start the day.

Quick Breakfast For People "On the go"

1. An apple and nuts (or cheese)
2. Grapes and nuts (or cheese)
3. Melon and nuts (or cheese)
4. Tuna, cheese and tomatoes
   on the side
5. Leftover vegetables
   (add cheese and heat)
6. Boiled eggs, cheese,
   fruit, vegetables

Have fun with the combinations. Just don't skip breakfast. When you do, you store your lunch and your dinner. The body is being told that you are starving and part of its job is to slow down the metabolic rate and conserve energy because the body does not know when you are going to feed it again. It does this to protect you. So you are not to skip any meals, for that simply invites trouble.

Lunch

Let's go back in time to early man. In the mid-portion of the day, he would go to the forest and the creeks, pick greens, berries and nuts and eat them on sight. There was no refrigerator. Everything was fresh, green, crisp and refreshing. Men would just eat what they needed and would come back daily to eat some more.

We have a primitive instinct passed down from our ancestors to chew something which is crunchy and green during the mid-portion of our day. That craving should be satisfied with a salad. Currently we are crunching on everything except a salad - croutons, chips, pretzels, crackers and candy bars.

Lunch is also a time for a protein source such as meat, eggs, soy, cheese, nuts and fruits. Always remember for lunch to select vegetables, protein and fruit. Eating fruit one hour after lunch will prevent fermentation or gas.

Caution: Eating a salad at dinner-time versus lunch prompts getting up in the middle of the night to urinate and this contributes to insomnia, restlessness, chronic fatigue and aging.

Whether you are having fast food or enjoying a fine dining experience for lunch, it's no big deal. Stay in control. Stop eating sandwiches. The bread takes three hours to digest, the meat takes six. However; when you combine the two, a chemical reaction takes places which slows down the digestion process and it takes up to fifteen hours to digest that sandwich. In the meantime, your metabolism crashes and you're nodding off during the early afternoon. That's when people start to raid the candy and soda machines. Getting sleepy or fatigued at this time of day contributes to weight gain.

When eating out this is how you should order: "I'll take the chicken sandwich. I'm refraining from bread, so please substitute extra lettuce and tomatoes." When you go through the line, leave the fries and soda and order water, juice or herbal tea.

If you're at a place of fine dining, order lemon with your water, send the bread basket back and substitute a side salad (take it home for tomorrow's lunch)! Substitute extra steamed vegetables for the rice pilaf, baked potato or corn which would raise your insulin level significantly at this time of day.

Have fruit, whipped cream and nuts for dessert. This has a beautiful presentation and is guaranteed to keep you on track.

Dinner

Dinner is quite simple. Eat your protein source (however you want it fixed) and two servings of vegetables. Here you can add a serving of complex carbohydrates. This means a serving of rice, pasta, potato or bread. Happy? I did not totally eliminate everything that we enjoy. I just put it in the right place. Guess what happens when you do this. One serving of complex carbohydrates does not sufficiently elevate the insulin level because this is the time to slow down, the time to rest. During the earlier part of the day we should not eat "resting" or "slow-down" foods because it is not time to rest.

The evening meal is a resting meal. When the complex carbohydrates are removed from breakfast and lunch, something wonderful happens. They become potent, like a sedative, and they help you to sleep! So much for insomnia.

Speaking of sleep, if you have chronic pain, restlessness, fatigue or insomnia, do not eat a salad with dinner or drink beverages after dinner. Why? It's called delayed water. This causes your bladder to become restless and it will keep you awake at night.

Eating like this suppresses the appetite. One serving of a complex carbohydrate is quite enough. The size of the servings will soon be half of what you are use to eating.

This program definitely saves money. The average family on my program has saved anywhere from $100 to $200 per month on their grocery bill. Conserving our food resource will enable us to have enough good food to feed our next generation.

<u>Snacks</u>

    -fruits
    -vegetables
    -protein sources

Again, I suggest you refer to Dr. D'Adamo's book "Eat Right For Your Type" to make the best selections.

<u>Desserts</u> - be creative

    -fruit
    -whipped cream
    -nuts

Bread Exception:

There is a high-protein, low-sodium bread that is good for all people regardless of their blood type. It does not significantly raise the insulin level as it is made with sprouted (unprocessed) ingredients. It is called Ezekiel 4:9 Bread. It is from the Bible:

"Take also unto thee wheat, and barley, and beans, and lentils, and millet, and spelt, and put them in one vessel, and make bread of it..." Ezekiel 4:9

This bread sustained the people referred to in the Bible verse for 390 days. They ate only the bread and drank water. It has been analyzed and has all the essential amino acids that sustains life.

Beverages

*Ice Water - the colder the better. The body must raise the temperature of the water to 98.6 degrees in order to absorb it; therefore, it's like doing an internal aerobic exercise.

*One glass of ice water actually burns off 120 calories!

*Lemon water or lemonade (not artificial) burns fats and lowers the insulin effect.

*Grapefruit juice is another great fat burner. Discuss with your doctor the absorption of certain medications before drinking large quantities.

*Herbal teas are healing teas. They are good for water retention, headaches, menstrual cramps, insomnia, libido, stress and much more.

RECAP OF FOOD CHOICES

BREAKFAST: fruit
                    vegetables
                    protein

LUNCH: salad
                    protein
                    fruit (one hour later)

DINNER: protein
                    2 cooked vegetables
                    1 carbohydrate
                    (Will not increase the insulin level when eaten at this time of day.)

SNACKS: fruit
                    vegetable
                    protein

BEVERAGES: ice water
                        lemon water
                        grapefruit
                        fruit juice
                        herbal tea

Note: Ideal meals will include lean meat, unsaturated fats and fiber.

Complex Carbohydrates:

rice (white)
corn
bread
beans
cereal
beets
carrots
potatoes (red/white)
bananas
pasta
soda
coffee
sugar
flour (white)

Fruits that burn fat:

kiwi
strawberry
blueberry
raspberry
boysenberry

pineapple
lemon
grapefruit
papaya
melons
plums

Protein Choices:

Meat

Soy

Cottage cheese

Yogurt

Nuts

*To get optimal results, choose foods, beverages and spices that are recommended for your blood group. You will now be on your way to diminishing, correcting and preventing many medical conditions; not only for yourself, but also for those you love and care about.

CHAPTER 4

Exercise At It's Best

Exercise

Recommendations from the American Heart Association, American Cancer society and the College of Obstetrics and Gynecology say that we all should exercise moderately 30 minutes, three time a week. Let's admit it, most people don't do that. Let me show you something real simple that anyone with any medical condition, any age, any size can do.

It starts in the bed: S-T-R-E-T-C-H

Stretching releases endorphins which are hormones that make you feel good all day! Endorphins also help burn peripheral fat. Can you imagine feeling good naturally everyday?

Lay flat in the bed on your back. Fan out your fingers, fan out your toes, suck in the abdomen and tighten the buttocks. Hold it for a count of ten. Do ten repetitions. Then do twenty repetitions. This strengthens the abdominal muscles and stimulates regular bowel movements.   People with tight abdomens have less incident of colon cancer and heart disease.   Good tone strengthens blood vessels and enables more oxygen to get to vital tissue and clear free radicals which cause disease and cancer.

Then ball up in the fetal position, squeeze the shoulders and squeeze the pelvis for a count of ten. Do ten repetitions. Then repeat on the other side. This brings blood to the pelvis.   In women, this enhances sexual response and strengthens the bladder. Vaginal and rectal muscles are also toned.   In men, it brings vital blood to the pelvis and enhances sexual response and gives better rectal control.

When you get out of bed and go the bathroom; as you sit on the toilet, swing your arms and legs in and out. This tones your inner and outer upper arms and the inner and outer thighs. While you brush you teeth move your legs (i.e. walking in place).

Driving affords an opportunity to alternately tighten and relax the pelvic muscles. This exercise is called Kegels. It also firms the buttocks and thighs.

Let's Add It All Up:

10 minutes of stretching
 4 minutes on the toilet
 6 minutes brushing teeth(am & pm)
20 minute driving commute
40 minutes everyday

Just imagine, forty minutes of exercise and no extra time was spent! There is no excuse. This is exercise at its best!

Always try to work in an additional thirty minutes of active or aerobic exercise. This could be walking, skating, running etc., three times a week. Any exercise that is done before breakfast mobilizes stored peripheral fat for its energy source. This is key. This will aid in maintaining your weight loss. If you have children, incorporate some exercise into their daily routine, including stretching.

Weight-lifting - Do it everyday

Don't panic. I'm not necessarily talking about bar bells and dumb bells. The current recommendation is that we weight-lift at least two times a week; however, we should do some form of weight-lifting everyday. Lift a can of food. Ladies, lift your purses. Lift until the arm or leg gets a burning sensation or lift to the point that you can no longer lift.

At that point, microfibers of muscle have just ruptured, to put it mildly. That however is good because after the first hour of sleep, the pituitary gland will release growth hormone to mend or repair the fiber. The growth hormone is you friend because it builds muscle, builds bone and most of all, it **suppresses aging**. Yes, I said aging. The growth hormone is the youth hormone and it retards the aging process as it plumps up dry aging cells. Remember the exercise guru Jack LaLaine? He never aged because he broke youth fiber everyday!

CHAPTER 5

Get Out of the Shower

Baths -vs- Showers

Showers are quick, fast and time efficient. We see more companies advertising shampoo products, for both skin and hair, in the shower versus the bath tub. Showers are stressful to the body as the water pelts, pulsates and pulverizes the skin. Stress raises the insulin level; therefore, showers can contribute to the rise of the insulin level and you know what that does to disease. Showers age the body!

As you look at TV and magazine ads depicting showers, remember what I explained about advertising, money and our health. We must safeguard ourselves from accepting information that leads us into unhealthy practices.

Let's look at nature. On the planet, do we have more waterfalls or more creeks, ponds, lakes, rivers or oceans? Let's look at animals. Do they bathe under waterfalls or in pools of water? Even looking at humans, our babies in the womb are in a pool of water. Taking a warm bath is like going back into your mother's womb where everything was quite peaceful, serene and soft. The tub is a place for reflection, meditation and prayer. This is why we must bathe.

We should bathe twice a day, especially in the morning to lower the insulin level for the day. We should also bathe in the evening prior to bedtime. The warm water induces relaxation and lowers the insulin as well as boosts the immune system. The insulin's lower level will guard and protect against cancer, hypertension, diabetes, angina, etc. while we sleep. Isn't that wonderful!

Brushing Is A Must

Before taking a bath, use a dry, long-handled, natural bristle brush on the entire dry body. Start at the feet and work your way up. Stroke each plane of the body about ten times each. Therefore, the legs should receive about 40 - 50 strokes. Brush gently upward away from gravity. After a dry brush preparation, a 30 minute bath using peppermint soap is highly recommended. Wonderful things are occurring now:

1. Brushing stimulates the immune system, the system that is responsible for protecting the body against stress, infections, arthritis, cancer, etc. Brushing lowers the insulin level.

2. Brushing can make varicose veins and spider veins fade and disappear after a period of time. The valves within the vessels improve their integrity and encourages the blood to return to the arteries.

3. Brushing improves the peripheral circulation; therefore, helps reduce swelling of the hands, ankles and feet. This also enhances the performance of the heart and supplies the body with more vital oxygen.

4. Brushing removes dead skin and leaves the body with the softness and glow of a

baby's bottom. Regular use helps remove skin moles and stretch marks.

Most exciting of all:

5.   Brushing stimulates the lymphatic channels. The heat from the water and the peppermint bath opens the skin pores, increases the body's peripheral circulation and releases the cellulite or stored fat and toxins through the skin and into the circulation and deposits it in the urine and the stool for elimination. Yes, there is help for cellulite; so run get those brushes!

CHAPTER 6

Let's Put It All Together

Fine Tuning

You now understand that there are certain foods that contribute to our illnesses and can speed our premature demise if we don't make some changes. I've outlined meals, snacks, exercise and skin care. Now let's fine tune a few things.

Before you get started, have a complete physical examination. Make sure you have your blood pressure, blood sugar, lipid profile, thyroid, blood type and any other pertinent laboratory values obtained. Women, make sure your pap smear test and mammograms are up-to-date. Men, you'll want to make certain you get a thorough prostate examination and have your Prostrate Specific Antigen (PSA) level checked to evaluate for cancer.

Studies have shown that according to your specific blood type (O, A, B, or AB), there are certain meats, certain vegetables, certain fruits, beverages, spices and even certain exercises that benefit your health. That is, they keep you from being obese, diabetic, hypertensive, depressed as well as keeping you from developing allergies, asthma, cancer or even having insomnia, thyroid problems and premature aging. And there of course are foods that do the complete opposite.

You should not put another morsel in you mouth until you know if you should be eating that particular food according to your blood type. Again, I highly recommend Dr. Peter D'Adamo's book "Eat Right 4 Your Type". It will complement the information you are reading here.

Once you incorporate this program and it becomes your lifestyle; for those seeking weight loss, you may stagnate or plateau at different points during the program. It's quite simple to remedy. Just increase your exercise, drink 8 glasses of ice water and for one week delete the fruits and vegetables choices from breakfast only. Insert an additional protein choice. After one week, go back to the fruits and vegetable choices and one protein choice for breakfast. Please don't forget that muscle weighs 22% more than fat. Therefore, as you become more physically active, you are indeed building muscle. Sometimes you will not see a significant drop on the scale right away or lose as quickly as you wish, but just hold on.

Do yourself a favor. Just try on a pair of tight pants (pants never lie), they will tell you if you are losing or not.

Remember, restoration takes time, preparation, support, passion and prayer. It may take you two months or it may take you two years to reach your goal. But as long as it is going in a positive direction you will see improvement and that's what you want. You want to be healthy. It's what we've all been looking for.

CHAPTER 7

Vitamins and Minerals

Since the foods we now eat are devoid of many of the nutrients that our great-grandparents had the benefit of, we must supplement our diet with vitamins and minerals. As always, please check with your physician or herbalist prior to starting anything new.

Female 18-30	Female 30-45	Female over 45
Multivitamin	Multivitamin	Multivitamin
Vit. C 1000 mg	Vit. C 1000 mg	Vit. C 1000 mg
	Chromium 200mg	Chromium 200mg
	Vitamin E 1000mg	Vitamin E 1000mg
		Calcium 1000mg
		Ginkgo Biloba

Male 18-30	Male 30-45	Male over 45
Multivitamin	Multivitamin	Multivitamin
Vit. C 1000 mg	Vit. C 1000 mg	Vit. C 1000 mg
	Chromium 200mg	Chromium 200mg
	Vitamin E 1000mg	Vitamin E 1000mg
		Calcium 1000mg
		Ginkgo Biloba

Children 0-18

Multivitamin
Vitamin C 500 mg

I recommend that you invest in a good book on herbs to help maintain good health. Ask your doctor about using herbs to supplement your treatment plan for any condition you may already be experiencing.

Multivitamins are loaded with vitamins and mineral which may contain the following list and the benefits derived from each:

Vitamin E - 1000mg
- decrease the severity of hot
  flashes
- decrease heart disease
- decrease prostate cancer
- decrease the symptoms of
  Alzheimer's
- antioxidant; cancer fighter
- restores skin moisture
- retards aging
- minimizes scar formation
  and tightening

Vitamin E rich foods: Vegetable oils, nuts, seeds, green leafy vegetables, liver
----

Calcium - 1000 mg
- builds bone
- retards osteoporosis
- improves nerve function

Calcium rich foods: green vegetables, nuts, seafood, dairy products

----

Vitamin C - 1000 mg

- diuretic
- restores cells
- promotes healing
- antioxidant
- builds collagen

Vitamin C rich foods: fruits, vegetables, meat, fish

Beta-Carotene - 25,000 IU

- antioxidant

Beta-Carotene rich foods: carrots, apricots, cantaloupe, spinach, broccoli

B Complex Vitamins: (water-soluble)
B1 - thiamin
B2 - riboflavin
B3 - niacin
B5 - pantothenic acid
B6 - pyridoxine
B12

The B Complex vitamins help reduce stress and the symptoms of anemia

Vitamin B rich foods: organ meat, seafood, eggs, cheese, nuts

----

SELENIUM - Antioxidant
- Immune booster
- retards aging
- decreases cholesterol

Selenium rich foods: meats, seafood, nuts

CHROMIUM
-improves insulin receptors'
 integrity
- builds lean muscle
- improves thyroid function
- helps the body burns fat

efficiently
- is depleted with exercise
Few foods offer significant amounts of chromium.

VITAMIN D - 400 IU
- builds bone

Vitamin D rich foods: diary products

IRON

- corrects anemia
- promotes wound healing

Iron rich foods: organ meats, green leafy vegetables

CHAPTER 8

Anoint Thyself With Oil

Essential oils have proven to be beneficial in obtaining and monitoring good health. The oils are concentrated and must be used with caution as they may irritate the skin. They may be diluted with either olive oil, jojoba oil, evening primrose oil, Vitamin E oil or Vitamin E cream.

Oil massage reduces stress, improves muscle tone, improves skin tone, boosts the immune system and improves circulation. The oils can be dispersed in a room with a room infuser or simply by placing an oil ring on a light bulb. It may also be put on cotton balls and placed in various areas in the room. A few drops can be added to the bath tub as a part of a therapeutic regimen. Following is a list of essential oils with their specific uses. Again, check with your physician or herbalist on the proper use of these products. Remember, keep oils out of the reach of children and check with your physician before using oils on children.

Anise - skin repair
Basil - arthritis, fatigue, depression

Bergamot- infection, herpes, depression, hair growth

Black currant - infection

Borage - skin regeneration

Calendula - skin

Camphor- trauma, calming, depression, analgesic, infection

Castor- detoxification of liver, digestive, gallbladder, laxative

Cedar wood - diuretic, calming, acne, oily skin, dandruff, hair growth

Chamomile - allergies, relaxation, neuralgia, dry skin, diarrhea, anemia, acne, depression, sleep, psoriasis, cramps, stress, cystitis, PMS, arthritis

Cinnamon- relaxation, infection

Cistus - calming

Citronella - insect repellent

Clary sage - relaxation, hair growth, skin, neuralgia, depression, hypertension, infection, cramps, libido, PMS

Clove - analgesic, relaxation, toothache

Coconut - skin

Cypress - cellulite

Dill - hypertension, stress, circulation

Eucalyptus - congestion, acne, allergies, herpes, neuralgia, cough, insect bites, cystitis, fungus, headaches

Evening primrose - hormonal balance, skin, arthritis, psoriasis

Fennel - digestion, cellulite, diuretic

Frankincense - cramps, cystitis, skin, stretch marks, nose bleeds, infection

Geranium - skin, circulation, cellulite, infection, hemorrhoids, liver, kidney, neuralgia, stress, PMS, cramps, diuretic, eczema

Ginger - nausea, digestion, circulation

Grape seed - tone skin, antioxidant

Hops - relaxation, sleep

Jasmine - sensual, relaxation, skin, depression, well-being

Jojoba - skin, restores hair growth

Juniper - circulation, acne, joint pain, cramps, digestion, urinary infection

Lavender - sleep, hair growth, eczema, acne, psoriasis, allergies, PMS, neuralgia, varicose veins, cystitis, herpes, memory, asthma, yeast, cellulite, stretch marks, cramps, hypertension, infections, diabetes, circulation, fungus, well-being, fatigue

Lemon - bronchitis, infection, fever, digestion, tones skin, oily skin, arthritis, hypertension, acne, laxative, anemia, varicose veins

Lemon balm - relaxation, sleep, anemia, hypertension,

Lemon grass - acne, hypertension, anemia

Lime - infection, digestion, tones skin

Lindon - relaxation

Melissa - relaxation, sleep

Myrrh - immunity, skin, infection, wound healing, yeast, hemorrhoids, fungus

Neen - infection

Neroli - skin

Orange - infection, immunity, skin

Patchouli - sensual, fever, nausea, wounds, diuretic, hair growth, cellulite, dandruff, depression, infection

Pennyroyal - infection, digestion, gas, circulation

Peppermint - relaxation, hair growth, sleep, memory, diarrhea, cough, psoriasis, cellulite, congestion, bronchitis, stimulation, muscle cramps, fever

Pine - sinus, joint pain, muscle pain

Rice bran - energy, reduces cholesterol

Rose - sensual, herpes, digestion, infection, skin, eczema, PMS, asthma, heart, liver

Rose hips - skin regeneration, diuretic

Rosemary - headaches, constipation, muscle pain, stress, gastritis, invigorating, arthritis, diuretic, dandruff, hair growth, lice, memory, fibromyalgia, multiple sclerosis, PMS, cellulite, circulation

Sandalwood - cough, allergies, sensual, calming, sleep, urinary tract infection, congestion, eczema

Sassafras - cleanser, gastritis

Spearmint - relaxation, simulates sleep, congestion, digestion

Spruce - invigorating

Tea tree - wounds, infection, herpes, fungus, fever, yeast, cystitis, lice, dandruff

Thyme - infection, deprecation, immune system, circulation, enemia, cough

Wheat germ - hot flashes, eczema, psoriasis, scars

Wintergreen-stimulates relaxation, infection, congestion

Ylang ylang - sensual, relaxation, oily skin, hypertension, hair growth, sleep, allergies, circulation

Buying Herbs and Oils

Choose a reputable manufacturer, not all are equal. Choose a store that has lots of business and turnover. This reduces the likelihood of extended shelf-life of its herbs and oils. Choose a store that has a knowledgeable staff. This makes a serious difference in your health status.

Talk to your doctor, herbalist or pharmacist about inter-actions, side effects, contraindications and indications. Follow instructions carefully.

Read the labels carefully. Purchase a good herb reference book to familiarize yourself with the herb, its use and its drawbacks. Use only as directed.

Discuss your physician any plan for using alternative medicine. Quite often herbs and oils may be used alone or in conjunction with traditional methods of treatment or therapy.

CHAPTER 9

Conditions and Diseases
and Their Remedies

The use of oils, herbs, foods, vitamins, massages, inhalants, teas and ointments have been used since the beginning of time to help people heal and maintain wellness. Again, I want to remind you to consult your physician or herbalist before you try anything new. There are many good reference books on the use of natural products. The following is just a sampling of conditions and diseases and the oils, herbs, foods, vitamins and minerals that are often found helpful.

ACNE - Chickweed, burdock, White oak bark, Echinacea, dandelion, aloe vera, cayenne, ginseng, valerian, chamomile, lavender, peppermint, juniper leaves, lemon grass, clary sage, tea tree, cedar wood, eucalyptus, geranium, Ylang ylang, sassafras, red clover, nettle, spinenard, beta carotene, vitamin B6, zinc, brewer's yeast

ATTENTION DEFICIT DISORDER - St. John's Wort, flax seed oil, primrose oil, magnesium, calcium, B-Complex, sandalwood, lavender, gingko biloba, Kava

Kava, stramonium, cina, gingko biloba, lemon balm, valerian, peppermint

AGE SPOTS- zinc, dandelion, selenium, calcium, gotu kola, bilberry, magnesium, Vitamin A, Vitamin E, Vitamin C, ginseng, licorice ginseng, sarsaparilla

AGING- ginseng, ginkgo biloba, omega-3 fatty acids, Vitamin E, Vitamin C, DHEA, peppermint, lavender, ylang ylang

ALCOHOLISM- Hops, passionflower

ALLERGIES - Ylang ylang, rose, sandalwood, lavender, eucalyptus, chamomile, goldenseal, peppermint.

ANEMIA - Lemon, chamomile, thyme

ARTHRITIS- cat's claw, cayenne, blessed thistle, juniper, chamomile, cypress, sage, lemon, thyme, zinc, primrose, ginger, rosemary, pine, eucalyptus, pineapple, celery, kale, garlic, alfalfa, Vitamin E, feverfew, mullein, omega-3 fatty acids,

DHEA, nettle, red clover, burdock, Vitamin C, ginkgo biloba, lavender

ASTHSMA/BRONCHITIS - Frankincense, rose, sweet marjoram, sandalwood

BED WETTING- Catnip, St. John's Wort, chamomile

BLOOD- red clover, yellow dock, sassafras, St. John's Wort

CANCER - kale, garlic, blueberry, blackberry, strawberry, DHEA, Vitamin C, Vitamin E, Vitamin A, carrot, celery, beet, clover, omega-3 fatty acids, selenium, echinacea, cat's claw, gotu kola, green tea, beta carotene, selenium, folate, zinc

CELLULITE - oregano, fennel, peppermint, rosemary, cypress, frankincense, lavender, neroli, geranium, jasmine, myrrh, chamomile, calenda, patchouli, grapefruit

CHOLESTEROL - red yeast, red clover, chickweed, lecithin, garlic, niacin, green tea

CHRONIC FATIGUE - bee pollen, rosemary, gingko biloba, lecithin, peppermint, lavender

CIRCULATION - juniper, hyssop, skullcap, peppermint, lemon balm, cypress, capsicum, ginger, ginkgo biloba, gotu kola, licorice, valerian, cayenne, goldenseal, white oak bark, tofu, black pepper, geranium, rosemary, ylang ylang

COLON CLEANSER - aloe, cascoia, sagrada, ginger, myrrh, psyllium, slippery elm, lemon

CONSTIPATION - buckthorn, cascara, sagrada, green barley, licorice, myrrh, psyllium, slippery elm, aloe, Vitamin C, rosemary, lemon

DANDRUFF - Rosemary, tea tree, cedarwood, patchouli

DEPRESSION/WELL BEING - blackberry, cherry, plum, skullcap, melissa, aspen, St. John's Wort, gotu kola, ignatia, ginseng, kava kava, feverfew, DHEA, selenium, chromium picolonate, camphor, fenugreek, ginkgo biloba, B-Complex, echinacea, chamomile, peppermint, lemon, lemon balm, lemon grass, jasmine, basil, thyme, bergamot, bee pollen, clary sage, rosemary, nutmeg, tangerine, ylang ylang, tea tree, ginger, selenium, Vitamin C, Vitamin E, astragalus, lavender, sandalwood, neroli, frankincense

DIABETES - licorice, dill, ylang ylang, geranium, fennel, ginger, hyssop, juniper, lavender, pine, rosemary, eucalyptus, raspberry, garlic, peppermint, green tea, chromium, Vitamin B, Vitamin C, Vitamin B12, zinc, potassium

DIARRHEA - chamomile, lavender, peppermint, eucalyptus

EDEMA - parsley, raspberry, dandelion, goldenseal, sarsaparilla, fennel, Vitamin C, fenugreek, blue cohosh, catnip, cornsilk, hops, gotu kola, horsetail, St. John's Wort, safflower, rosemary, chamomile, geranium, lemon, lemon grass

ENERGIZER- astragalus, ginseng, rosemary, gotu kola, peppermint

FEVER - alfalfa, nettle, vervain, white oak, yarrow, tea tree, peppermint, lemon, rosemary

FIBROMYALGIA or MULTIPLE SCLEROSIS - raspberry, rosemary, ginger, pine, eucalyptus, fungus, milkweed pod, juniper, thyme, chamomile, lavender, geranium, clary sage

GAS - angelica, wild yam

GASTRITIS - peppermint, chamomile, ginger, angelica, bromelain, fennel, fenugreek, skullcap, uva-ursi, agrimony, licorice, bilberry, omega-3 fatty acids, garlic, cabbage, carrot, celery, psyllium, flax seed, licorice, lavender, rosemary, clary sage, rose, frankincense

GOUT - garlic, kale, bromelain, sarsaparilla, yucca, peppermint, lavender

HAIR, NAILS - horsetail, jojoba, kelp, sarsaparilla, yucca, flax seed, omega-3 fatty acids, garlic, magnesium, beta carotene, calcium, lecithin, bee pollen, saw palmetto, ginseng, rosemary, sage, Vitamin C, Vitamin B6, walnut leaves, peppermint, coconut, pandanus leaf, fenugreek, sandalwood, cinnamon, aloe vera, chamomile, lavender, clary sage, cedarwood, patchouli, ylang ylang, rose, geranium.

HEADACHES - lavender, peppermint, eucalyptus, sweet marjoram, rosemary

HEART - angelica, hawthorn, licorice, ginkgo biloba, Vitamin E, Vitamin C, Vitamin B6, DHEA, carrot, beet, calcium, magnesium, garlic, chromium, lecithin, lavender, ylang ylang, rosemary, cayenne, lemon, cypress, gotu kola, juniper, ginger, goldenseal, rose

HEMORRHOIDS - aloe, cascara, sagrada, frankincense, geranium, juniper

HERPES - echinacea, Vitamin C, lysine, dandelion, astragalus, goldenseal, passion flower, raspberry, tea tree, eucalyptus, bergamot, lemon, lavender

HOT FLASHES - Vitamin E, black cohosh, damicana, don quai, wild yam, evening primrose, sage, horsetail, ginseng, hawthorn, licorice, Vitamin C, DHEA, omega-3 fatty acids, lavender, chamomile, rose

HYPERTENSION - lavender, peppermint, ylang ylang, clary sage, chamomile, garlic, capsicum, dandelion, hawthorn, parsnip leaves, flax seed, calcium, magnesium, potassium, niacin, carrot, celery, beet, asparagus, brown rice, green tea, lemon, sweet marjoram

IMMUNITY - peppermint, echinacea, goldenseal, pau d'arco, DHEA, selenium, Vitamin C, zinc, elderberry,

INSECTS - citronella, pennyroyal, tea tree, eucalyptus, geranium, chamomile, lemon, lemon grass

INSOMNIA - peppermint, chamomile, passion flower, valerian, hawthorn, hops, rose, kava kava, skullcap, geranium, lavender, sweet marjoram, orange, sandalwood, ylang ylang

IRREGULAR MENSES - St. John's Wort

KIDNEY - lecithin, nettle, sheep sorrel, slippery elm, white oak, agrimony, fenugreek

LICE - tea tree, rosemary

LIVER - milk, thistle, sassafras, fennel, feverfew, hops, ho show wir, fenugreek, garlic

MUSCLE/MENSTRUAL CRAMPS - basil, chamomile, peppermint, parsley, jasmine, clary sage, lavender, cypress, bergamot, rosemary, cayenne, eucalyptus, black cohosh, raspberry, feverfew, geranium, frankincense, sweet marjoram

MIGRAINES- fenugreek, feverfew, thyme, raspberry, parsley

NAUSEA - peppermint, tea tree, lavender, grapefruit, rose, juniper, rosemary, sandalwood, fennel

OBESITY - Selenium, chromium, sea wrack, bromelain, fennel, nettle, lecithin, kelp, buchu, cornsilk, hawthorn, burdock, DHEA, bee pollen, peppermint, lavender

OSTEOPOROSIS- calcium, broccoli

PMS - clary sage, lavender, chamomile, rosemary, geranium, rose, sweet marjoram

PROSTATE - saw palmetto, bee pollen, cornsilk, zinc, tofu, green tea, pygeum bark, goldenseal, desert tea, gingko biloba, lavender, peppermint

PSORIOSIS - lavender, chamomile, peppermint, tea tree

RESPIRATORY - eucalyptus, peppermint, pine, tea tree, sandalwood, rosemary, lavender, basil, ginger, goldenseal, hyssop, echinacea, mullein, thyme, vervain, yarrow, feverfew, bee pollen, Vitamin C, omega-3

fatty acids, frankincense, rose, lemon, lemon grass

SEXUAL - patchouli, ylang ylang, jasmine, sandalwood, yohimke, lavender, clary sage

SINUSITIS - blue violet, peppermint, coltsfoot, myrrh, spinenard, echinacea, goldenseal, thyme, vervain, sandalwood

STRESS - peppermint, lavender, clary sage, chamomile, geranium, rosemary

STRETCH MARKS - frankincense, lavender, neroli, geranium, patchouli

THYROID - kelp

URINARY TRACT - raspberry, buchu, cranberry, cornsilk, goldenseal, Uva-ursi, Vitamin C, chamomile, frankincense, tea tree, eucalyptus, lavender, geranium

VARICOSE VEINS - white oak bark, peppermint, lavender, horse chestnut, gotu kola, bromelain, grape seed, buckwheat, pine bark, blueberries, raspberries, Vitamin C, Vitamin E, lemon, lemon grass

VISION - bilberry, ginkgo biloba, eyebright, hyssop, kale, carrot, parsley, omega-3 fatty acids, cayenne, Vitamin A, spinach, tomato

WARTS - dandelion, lavender, peppermint

WRINKLES - lavender, lemon, lemon grass, lemon balm, frankincense

WOUNDS - aloe vera, chamomile, chickweed, echinacea, goldenseal, cayenne, dandelion, myrrh, horsetail, papaya, sage, garlic, slippery elm, St. John's Wort, valerian, white oak yucca, Vitamin E, tea tree, geranium, lemon, ylang ylang, frankincense

YEAST - echinacea, garlic, white oak, cayenne, goldenseal, tea tree, myrrh, lavender, eucalyptus

CHAPTER 10

Guidelines For Good Health

GUIDELINES FOR GOOD HEALTH

Guidelines For Children
Guidelines For Adults
Breast Self-Examination
Testicular Self-Examination
Pregnancy
Menopause
Smoking
Smog, dust and chemical exposure
Travel
Work Environment
Fiber
Fruit Facts
Party Food Guide
Natural Therapies
Health, Wellness & Restoration Summary

KEYS TO GOOD HEALTH

GUIDELINES FOR CHILDREN

Type of Service	Age Group	Check How Often
Medical History/ Physical	0-2 years 2-18 years	2, 4, 6, 9, 12, 15, & 18 months annually
Hepatitis B	0-2 years	birth, 2 months & 6-18 months
DTP	0-2 years	2, 4, 6 months & 15-18 months
TD booster	14-16 years	once, then every 10 years
H. influenzae	0-2 years	2, 4, 6 months & 15-18 months
Polio -booster	0-2 years 4-6 years	2, 4, 6 months
MMR -booster	0-2 years 4-6 years or 11-12 years	12-15 months
Chicken pox	0-2 years 11-12 years	12-18 months if no prior vaccination or history
Vision exam	4-18 years	annually
Hearing test	4-18 years	every 3 years
Hemoglobin/ Hematocrit	0-4 years	one time
Blood pressure	3-18 years	annually
Lead test	0-18 years	per doctor
Cholesterol	4-18 years	every 3 years

GUIDELINES FOR ADULTS

Type of Service	Age Group	Check How Often
Medical History/ Physical	19-99 years	annually
TD booster	19-99 years	every 10 years
MMR	19-99 years	per doctor
Influenza	19-65+ years	per doctor
Pneumonia	19-65+ years	per doctor
Hepatitis B	19-65+ years	per doctor
Vision exam	19-99 years	every 2 years
Hearing test	19-99 years	every 5 years
Rectal exam/ Hemocult	19-99 years	annually
Blood pressure	19-99 years	annually
Cholesterol	19-65+ years	every 3 years
Clinical & Self Breast Exams	19-99 years	annually
Mammogram	40-99 years	annually
Pap Smear	19-99 years	annually
Sigmoidoscopy	40-99 years	every 3-5 years
Bone Density	50-99 years	every 3 years
PSA	40-99 years	annually

1
While in the shower,

ise your right arm. Use the finger
nds of your left hand to touch every
art of your right breast. Feel gently
r any lumps or changes under the skin.
hen raise your left arm and use your
ght hand to examine your left breast.

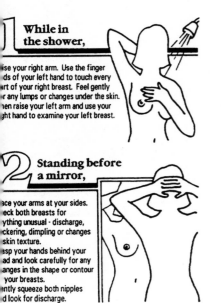

2
Standing before a mirror,

ace your arms at your sides.
eck both breasts for
ything unusual - discharge,
ckering, dimpling or changes
skin texture.
asp your hands behind your
ad and look carefully for any
anges in the shape or contour
your breasts.
ntly squeeze both nipples
d look for discharge.

3
Lie flat on your back,

with your left arm over your
head and a pillow or towel under
your left shoulder. Put your left
hand behind your head. Use your
right hand to begin touching
your left breast gently but firmly.

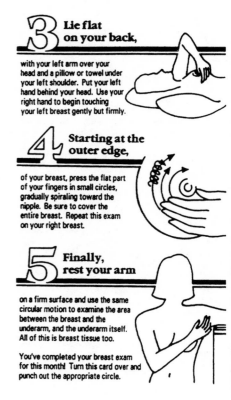

4
Starting at the outer edge,

of your breast, press the flat part
of your fingers in small circles,
gradually spiraling toward the
nipple. Be sure to cover the
entire breast. Repeat this exam
on your right breast.

5
Finally, rest your arm

on a firm surface and use the same
circular motion to examine the area
between the breast and the
underarm, and the underarm itself.
All of this is breast tissue too.

You've completed your breast exam
for this month! Turn this card over and
punch out the appropriate circle.

Testicular Self-Exam (TSE)

A simple 3 minute self-examination, once a month, can detect one of the cancers most common among men aged 15-34. If detected early, testicular cancer is one of the most easily cured.

The best time to check yourself is in the shower or after a warm bath. Fingers glide over soapy skin making it easier to concentrate on the texture underneath. The heat causes the skin to relax, making the exam easier.

1. Start by examining your testicles. Slowly roll the testicle between the thumb and fingers, applying slight pressure. Try to find hard, painless lumps.

2. Now examine your epididymis. This comma-shaped cord is behind each testicle. It may be tender to the touch. It's also the location of the most non-cancerous problems.

3. Continue by examining the vas (the sperm-carrying tube that runs up from your epididymis). The vas normally feels like a firm, movable smooth tube.

Now repeat the exam on the other side.

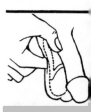

What are the symptoms?

In early stages testicular cancer may be symptomless. When symptoms do occur they include:

- Lump on the testicle
- Slight enlargement of one of the testes
- Heavy sensation in testicles or groin
- Dull ache in lower abdomen or groin

If you find any hard lumps or nodules, see your doctor promptly. Only your doctor can make a diagnosis.

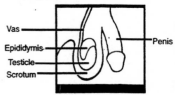

Vas —
Epididymis —
Testicle —
Scrotum —
Penis

"This self-exam is not a substitute for periodic examinations by a qualified physician."

"Bay Pacific Health Plan, 1988"

116

Pregnancy

Any woman who is attempting to become pregnant should see an obstetrician prior to conceiving for an updated physical, pap smear, mammogram and possible lab work. Have a rubella titer if the status is not known or perhaps a blood sugar or a thyroid panel if necessary.

The College of Obstetrics and Gynecology also recommends a prenatal supplement which contains 1 mg of folic acid. Folic acid supplements of 1 mg decreases the incidence of neuro tube defects by as much as 50%. The basic restorative program works quite well. Milk, yogurt, cheese or a calcium supplement should supply approximately 1,500 mg of total calcium per day. Snacks of fruit, vegetables and protein are encouraged.

You should avoid salads at dinner because of the delayed water phenomenon. In other words, you'll spend you night visiting the bathroom. You'll also want to stop drinking all fluids around 7:00 pm for the same reason.

As far as exercising is concerned, the exercises in the restorative program can easily be mastered by pregnant women. Walking, swimming and low impact aerobic exercise are also recommended. I strongly discourage high impact aerobics, running, skating and extremely strenuous exercises because of the threat of miscarriage or pre-term labor.

You'll love the brushing and bathing. My patients brush and bathe in peppermint baths twice a day. Their skin glows, their energy is optimal, they sleep well, they rarely are edematous. Not only do the mothers-to-be benefit from this restoration program, their babies are born extremely healthy.

Please discuss this program with your OB/GYN before starting so that he/she may make any modifications for your personal needs.

Menopause

Menopause (the stopping of menses) is that period of a woman's life cycle where you may undergo some physical and mental changes.

Menopause may occur naturally where the bleeding stops on its own or it may be prompted surgically following a hysterectomy. Some women have symptoms due to the significant decrease in the ovaries' hormone level of estrogen and progesterone. You may experience a few or a multitude of symptoms such as irregular uterine bleeding, hot flashes, cold flashes, night sweats, excessive perspiration, vaginal dryness, urinary burning, urinary irritation, vaginal bleeding, vaginal itching, decreased interest in sex or libido.

Women complain of water retention, weight gain, body aches and pains, hair thinning, dry skin, mood swings, memory loss and insomnia.

All of these symptoms can be decreased by following the Health, Wellness and Restoration Program with the addition of some foods, herbs and oils that help the menopausal woman. Remember to incorporate weight bearing exercises into your routine. This builds bone, muscles and release growth hormones which retard the aging process.

SUGGESTED MENOPAUSAL SUPPPLEMENTS:

Multivitamins
Vitamin E - 1000 mg
Vitamin C - 1000 mg
Calcium/Magnesium 1000 mg
Evening Primrose oil
Black cohosh
Blue cohosh
Garlic
Wild Yam Root
Citrus Fruits
Ginkgo Biloba
Green Tea
Lavender oil after bath
Progesterone

Ladies, you don't have to suffer. Nor do you have to rely solely on prescription remedies. You have many choices and options. Read books, clip articles, take notes, talk to your physician and be flexible.

You are only at the half way mark of your life's journey. Perhaps the better half!

Smoking

We know that smoking costs this country billions of dollars in health-related expenses, loss of work hours due to illness, disability and death. Most people would quit if they could, but they can't.

The benefits of being a non-smoker include:
* improved energy
* decrease in instances of:
    asthma
    bronchitis
    emphysema
    heart disease
    hypertension
    stroke
    tooth and gum disease
    cancer
    second-hand exposure
* reduced aging
* increased fertility

Smoking robs the cells of vital oxygen and Vitamin C. The latest studies have proved that smoking may contribute to newborns having cancer.

It's best to discuss the problem with your physician. There are many programs available; including group sessions, individual sessions, patches, acupuncture, behavior modification techniques, chewing gum and oral capsules. Just stay positive and focused. Alter your diet by removing the complex carbohydrates from the breakfast and lunch choices. You should increase exercise and drink plenty of ice water.

Wash the harmful pollutants of smoking from the skin before retiring. Remember, the skin, the largest organ of the body, is a sponge. It takes in everything. Avoid smoking around other people; it's the right thing to do.

Smog, Dust and Chemical Exposure

Smoke, smog, dust and fumes from chemicals are air born contaminates that can cause a multitude of illnesses. They all contain free radicals which are highly charged atoms that can alter normal cells into abnormal cells which cause diseases such as heart attacks, strokes, arthritis, asthma, bronchitis, emphysema, depression and cancer.

If you are exposed to these conditions, it is be crucial that you take therapeutic peppermint baths to remove toxic residue, apply lavender oil and drink lots of water to flush your system. The restorative program will keep you healthy in the face of these adverse conditions.

Travel

How many times can you remember getting sick while you are away from home; whether it was a business trip or vacation? I'm talking about headaches, migraines, upset stomach, constipation, joint pain, allergies, swelling of the feet and legs or insomnia. Traveling is stressful to the body. Stress, again, causes insulin to rise and that causes the whole cascade of diseases and problems to occur! So how do we avoid stress on trips, whether business or pleasure?

*Plan ahead. Pack leisurely; arrive early.

*Stretch and do deep breathing exercises once you get settled.

*Don't sit for long periods of time. Stretch and walk.

*Drink water instead of alcohol, soda or coffee.

*For calming, drink herbal teas - peppermint and chamomile.

*Drink raspberry teas or take fennel capsules to avoid swelling.

*Snack on fruits, nuts and vegetables. Avoid salty foods.

*Put peppermint lotion behind the ears and on the temples for calming.

*Use candles or infusers for aromatherapy.

*Tea tree oil is an excellent antiseptic.

*Use massage oils everyday.

*Listen to classical, soft jazz or new age music.

*Brush the skin and take peppermint baths each morning and night. Avoid showers if possible. Use lavender at night and rosemary in the morning.

*Zinc helps the immune system as does echinacea. Zinc is also good for a sore throat.

*Melotonin, lavender, valerian root, passion flower, chamomile and peppermint all help to promote sleep.

*Write letters. Read positive books.

*Avoid negative people and negative conversations.

You will return from your trip rested and relaxed!

Work Environment

Quite often you cannot control your work environment as far as the physical surroundings. However; you may be in a situation where you can alter your environment. Anytime you can control or at least influence the physical makeup of your work station or office, you can relieve some stress and express some creativity. By doing so, you reduce your blood insulin level and reduce the possibility of illness and disease.

Some suggestions:

-Arrive early. It tremendously reduces stress.

-Stretch and deep breathe once you get settled.

-Aromatherapy- use infusers and/or potpourri.

-Green plants put oxygen in the air.

-Flowers help calm you and beautify a room.

-Soft colors on walls and furniture; hang calming pictures.

-Family photos - the reason you work.

-Classical, soft jazz and new age music calms the spirit.

-Pack your lunch - relieves stress of deciding and buying.

-Walk outside. Get some fresh air and sunshine.

-Drink cold water. It burns off 120 calories per glass.

-Drink herbal teas - peppermint and chamomile are calming.

-Drink raspberry tea - relieves swelling.

-Snack on fruits, vegetables and proteins. Avoid salty foods.

FIBER FIBER FIBER

Not enough can be said about fiber. We are simply not getting enough dietary fiber in the present "good ole American diet". The recommended consumption of fiber is 30-35 grams per day. In third world countries, where the incidence of obesity, heart disease and cancer is low, many residents consume 60 grams of fiber per day.

People who have diets low in fiber have more incidences of obesity, heart disease, hypertension, diverticular disorders, gastrointestinal disorders, hemorrhoids, cancer and more. Fiber is that portion of our food that cleans the intestinal tract. Keeping the intestinal tract clean eliminates poisons and toxins more quickly and the incidence of disease drops dramatically.

Fiber supplements are very helpful in adding fiber to the diet without the addition of excess calories; which aids weight reduction.

Good sources of fiber:

Bran
Cabbage
Nuts
Pears
Carrots
Kidney Beans
Apples
Asparagus
Pinto Beans
Kiwi

Poor sources of fiber

Meat	Pasta
Fish	Wheat Bread
Dairy	Bananas

ALL FRUITS HAVE POTASSIUM

Fruit	Potassium	Carbohydrate	Calories
Kiwi	480	24	100
Banana	400	29	110
Nectarine	300	16	70
Cherry	300	22	90
Melons	280	12	50
Strawberries	270	12	45
Grapes	270	24	90
Orange	260	26	70
Grapefruit	230	32	120
Watermelon	230	27	80
Plums	220	19	80
Pears	210	25	100
Peaches	190	10	40
Apples	170	22	80
Tangerines	150	15	50
Pineapples	115	16	60
Lemons	90	5	15

*Potassium listed in milligrams
*Carbohydrates listed in grams

APPROVED PARTY FOODS

FOOD

Chicken Salad: cubed, cooked chicken with onion, garlic, mayo, celery and spices to taste (salt and pepper)

Tuna Salad: tuna, celery, onion, mayo, relish, eggs (optional)

Egg Salad: eggs, celery, onions, mayo, relish

Ham Salad: ground ham, eggs, relish, mayo

Tossed Salad or 7-Layer Salad

Deviled Eggs: toppings can include olives (black/green) & shrimp

Celery: cut into 4-5" pieces, stuff with cream cheese or peanut butter

Cheese tray

Pickle/Relish/Olive tray

BEVERAGES

Ice Water - add lemon wedges

Lemonade- sweetened/unsweetened

Iced Tea- sweetened/unsweetened

Herbal Tea- sweetened/
unsweetened

DESSERTS

Any fruit
Whipping cream
Nuts

CONDIMENTS

Lemon
Sweet & Low
Hot Sauce
Salt
Pepper
Olives
Pickles

FOODS TO AVOID

Soda
Coffee
Crackers
Cakes
Cookies
Bread
Potato chips
Bananas

NATURAL THERAPIES

There are many natural methods to increase and maintain good health. As always, consult with your physician before starting any new routine.

AROMATHERAPY: This is the case of essential oil in the air via a transfuser, on a light bulb or on a cotton ball. Aromatherapy is used for relaxation, healing or invigoration.

MASSAGE: This can be done in many ways. By a therapist or self massage using a vibrator or a soft bristle brush.

REFLEXOLOGY: There are certain areas of the feet which directly correspond to specific areas of the body. Applying various levels of pressure can help relax the body and promote healing.

HYDROTHERAPY: The body is submerged in a water tank with deprivation of all sound. It mimics the peace and calmness of a fetus in the uterus. The bathtub works great.

CHIROPRACTIC: Since 1885, chiropractic methods have been used in this country. It incorporates the use of special exercise, herbs, with emphasis on adjusting the spinal cord and soft body tissue. It concentrates on the nervous system.

HOMEOPATHY: This is the use of natural agents already found in the body to trigger the body to use its own defense mechanism to heal itself.

FEN SHUI: Involves creating a room or even a whole house that combines color, style, aromatherapy and other dynamics to fill one's specific lifestyle. The space would be arranged to promote peacefulness, relaxation, well being and creativity.

REIKI: Is a healing touch technique from Japan that emphasizes the rebirth of the body. It promotes healing by detoxifying the body.

MINERAL BODY WRAPS: The body is wrapped with natural gauze and minerals for two hours. This promotes a breakdown of peripheral body toxins that build up in the fat layer. Six to ten inches can be lost in one session.

MUD BATHS: These are quite popular in California. The minerals extract toxins from the fat layer and promotes well being.

ACUPUNCTURE: With origins from the Far East, acupuncture involves the insertion of fine needles that stimulate the nerve roots of specific areas of the body. This triggers the release of pain or depression. It is also used for anesthesia.

YOGA: An ancient practice of flexing the joints in a relaxed, calm setting. Meditation is a key component.

TAI CHI: Involves relaxation, stretching, focus and meditation.

DEEP BREATHING: This helps promote relaxation. Deep breathing builds red blood cells which in turns delivers more oxygen and nutrients to the body.

Testimonials

"I went on your health, wellness and restoration program completely. I am 72 years old. My knees were weak and now that is gone. My congestion is eliminated. The cramp from a pinched nerve is feeling diminished. Walking causes no more leg stress. I received a deep cut on my toe and it clotted right away."

-J.B., retired

"I am a 44 year-old physician. In two months I have gone from 175 pounds to 163; changed a shirt size and several belt notches. For the first time in two years, I've been able to put my wedding band on."

-M.D., Family Practice

"Being pregnant for the second time, I was dreading having the edema that I had with the first pregnancy. Dr. Davis suggested that I increase my intake of water and stop drinking soda. Within a week I noticed a difference. My swelling decreased and I found my skin feeling healthier."

-P.P., 32 year-old receptionist

"Since starting her diet, I have lost pounds and inches, increased my energy level and most of all, bettered my self-image and confidence."

-K.P., 26 year-old City employee

"For several years I have weighed between 185 and 199 lbs. I felt very poor. So I decided [that] I would [eat] low fats and low carbohydrates and fruit three times a day. From March to June, I lost 35 lbs. and I felt great. When my family doctor took my bloodwork, I was able to go off my blood pressure and cholesterol medicine and my thyroid was normal. My diabetes is now controlled by eating naturally and walking."

-I.M., 70 years old, retired

"I see a big difference with the brushing with a soft bristle brush before bathing. The spider veins have disappeared and I wear shorts with a smile."

-L.R., 41 year old cafeteria worker

"For several years I have weighed 247 lbs. I was unable to walk very far, for I had arthritis in my legs and feet. Everyday I would take over 4000 mg of aspirin just to be able to work. I would also have to take blood pressure medicine. I decided that I needed to do something about my weight. I started watching my fat and carbohydrate intake. Within a week, I started losing weight and I noticed I was walking better. Within a year's time, I was able to lose 107 lbs. From February to April, I was able to lose another 37 lbs and keep it off.

Since April, I have been able to keep my weight at 110 lbs. Also, I have worn glasses since 1973 and hearing aids since 1995. I now only wear my glasses to drive, watch TV and [to] see things far off. I do not wear my hearing aids at all. I have lost 137 lbs and I was flabby. With brushing twice a day and bathing in peppermint soap, I am just as firm as when I was a teenager. My husband and I walk at least three miles a day."

-J.M., 44 year old receptionist

"In December, 1997, my weight was 207 lbs. Now in July, 1998, I am 170 lbs. My fibroids have improved, my cholesterol is down as well as my blood pressure. I feel like I have decreased my age by 10 years and I can even get in my daughter's clothes, who is 16 years old."

-V.J., 41 year old business owner

"Diabetes and being overweight are issues that are prevalent in my family. At 5'2", I had gotten up to 160 [lbs] at one point. Now I'm down to 140 [lbs] and am still on my way. my thighs and legs are toned and sculpted. I use to wear a size 14, now I'm the proud owner of size 10 pants and skirts! My waistline shrunk, my energy level went through the roof and my appetite decreased. My skin cleared up and my hair is strong and thick."

-R.C., 30 year-old news anchor

"I am more confident and happier than I have ever been in my life. I have been fighting my weight since college. I believe that my constant weight fluctuations contributed to my lack of career advancement with my current employer of 17 years. I started with your system on January 21, 1998 and I weighed 256 pounds. Eight weeks later I was down to 228 pounds. I dropped a whole suit size! I now weigh 221 pounds and I am only 5 pounds away from my personal goal of 216 pounds.

my confidence soared and so did my performance on the job. I interviewed for a promotion and I got it!!"

R.C. 38 year-old pharmaceutical rep.

CHAPTER 11

Quick Tips and Program Recap

-Remember, the turtle won the race.

-Slow weight loss establishes good habits.

-Read labels for nutritional information.

-Water is calorie free.

-Exercise while you watch TV.

-Serve your plate from the stove.

-Place a water pitcher on the table.

-Drink 6 to 8 glasses of water a day.

-No beverage intake after 7:00 p.m.

-For insomnia, no salad with dinner.   This causes delayed urination.

-Order half-portions at restaurants.

-Send the bread basket away from the table.

-Substitute a salad for the bread basket.

-Order lemon wedges for the water.

-Use smaller dinner plates.

-Avoid second and third helpings.

-Share a dessert instead of ordering one for yourself.

-Order fruit for dessert instead of pie or cake.

-Substitute a vegetable for the complex carbohydrate.

-Steam cauliflower, cut it up and use for a rice substitute.

-Steam spaghetti squash as a pasta substitute.

-Fish for breakfast suppresses the appetite more than any other food.

-Apples and nuts - a quick, on-the-run meal or snack.

-Herbal eye mask promotes sleep.

-Quality sleep strengthens the immune system.

-Quality sleep retards aging.

-Relaxing the body decreases disease.

-Smoking decreases Vitamin C.

-Crash diets cause fatigue, muscle wasting and depression.

-Don't skip meals - you'll store the next two meals.

-If you snack, keep it healthy with fruit, vegetables or protein.

-Exercise before breakfast - mobilizes stored fat as energy base.

-Insist on healthy food in the workplace - your second home.

-Take your own food to social functions whenever permissible.

-Avoid smoking atmosphere - robs cell of vital oxygen.

-Stop eating when you are satisfied.

-If you want complex carbohydrates, always eat them with dinner.

-Turn down alcoholic beverages, drink water, tea or juice. Lite beer and dry red wine will keep you on the program.

-Keep your social and business schedule under control - reduces stress.

-Just say no! Sometimes enough is enough.

-Avoid complex carbohydrates in the morning and early day hours, they slow the metabolism.

-Muscle weighs more than fat.

-Save $100 to $200 per month on your food bill.

-Nicotine and caffeine increase urinary tract infections.

-A twenty pound weight gain increases the risk of breast cancer 40%.

-Fish decreases the risk of all cancers.

-Exercising 4 hours a week cuts breast cancer risk by 37%.

-Sunshine decreases breast cancer risk due to Vitamin D.

-Olive oil use decrease breast cancer risk.

-Smile! You'll feel so much better immediately.

-Fruits and vegetables are the best sources of fiber.

-35 grams of fiber per day is necessary for good health - Americans average 12 grams.

-Kegels help prevent hemorrhoids and enhance sexual response.

-Tight clothes contribute to edema.

-Mulitvitamins are a must. Our food is vitamin and mineral deficient.

-All fruits contain potassium

-We consume seven times the amount of salt than our ancestors did.

-Bread and pasta are only 10,000 years old - we're older.

-Over 60% of the American diet is food not eaten by our ancestors.

-Fish contains omega fatty acids - these prevent cancer.

-The fats from meats are good fats and designed for our bodies.

-Stress releases Vitamin C from the body - this decreases immunity.

-Mercury in tooth fillings contributes to fibromyalgia and multiple sclerosis.

-Butter is better than margarine.

-Vitamin E, Vitamin C and beta-carotene antioxidants reduce cholesterol.

-Don't depend on food for comfort.

-Do our family gatherings have to be so food-oriented?

-Garlic lowers cholesterol.

-Free radicals, which are oxidized or altered atoms, destroy collagen - they are neutralized by antioxidants.

-Melatonin, an antioxidant, helps insomnia.

-Dandelion invigorates and purifies; a great diuretic.

-Citronella keeps insects away.

-Massage reduces free radicals and therefore aging, cancer and heart disease.

-Massage boosts the immune system.

-Vitamin C, garlic and cranberry products help fight urinary infections.

-Antioxidants reduce Alzheimer's, cataracts, heart disease, cancer and aging.

-Free radicals are released by pesticides, smoke, radiation and sun exposure.

-Use sunscreen, at least SPF 15, on all exposed surfaces of the skin.

-Wear hats and sunglasses for eye and skin protection.

-Get a complete check-up by your physician every year.

-Always warm up before strenuous activity and cool down afterward.

-Vitamin E boosts collagen and retards aging.

-Sleep between 7 -8 hours a night.

-Vitamin E retards aging, restores cells and moisturizes the skin.

-Vitamin E retards heart disease, hot flashes, prostate cancer and Alzheimer's.

-Weight-lifting releases growth hormones; which retards aging.

-Alternate your exercise program for the best yield.

-Stop sugar ingestion to stop cravings.

-Packaged broccoli has more Vitamin C than unpackaged broccoli.

-Salmon, tuna and sardines are rich in omega-3 fatty acids.

-Eat 5-8 servings of fruits and vegetables a day.

-Acupuncture helps relieve poor skin tone.

-For better sleep, avoid caffeine, alcohol and cigarettes.

-Women lose one-third pound of muscle weight per year after age 40.

-Peppermint boosts alertness and mental ability.

-Peppermint is a natural anti-bacterial herb.

-Peppermint helps stop the itch of insect bites.

-Breathing from the diaphragm puts oxygen in the blood.

-Learn some self-massage techniques.

-Switch from caffeinated to decaf beverages.

-Sodas have no nutritional value.

-Coffee has no nutritional value.

-Strive for 35 grams of fiber per day.

-Monounsaturated fats include avocado, nuts, olive and canola oils.

-Your blood type determines your reaction to diseases.

-Three to four eggs a week are safe.

-Eating foods high in natural estrogen retards Alzheimer's disease.

-During the first six years after menopause, a woman loses one-third of her spinal bone mass.

-Red peppers are higher in Vitamin C than green peppers.

-Exercise helps control insomnia.

-Pink grapefruit has more beta carotene than white grapefruit.

-Snow peas have more calcium than green peas.

-Romaine has more Vitamin C and beta carotene than iceberg lettuce.

-Speed up ripening of tomatoes by placing them in a bag with an apple.

-Smoked turkey is used more and more to season greens and green beans.

-Herbs and spices are used more and more to season greens and green beans.

-Complex carbohydrates increase serotonin and tryptophan, therefore these reduce stress.

-Magnesium regulates serotonin, helps headaches and PMS.

-Herbs are 65% more effective than traditional medicines.

-Love handles are fat deposits over the oblique muscles.

-Women store fat in the lower abdomen and thighs.

-Wash the back of the hands, between the fingers and under the nails.

-If a person is 20% overweight, their LDL levels are elevated.

-Proteins are composed of oxygen, carbon, hydrogen and nitrogen.

-Carbohydrates contain not nitrogen, therefore cannot build and repair.

-Most people want optimal health the most natural way.

-Dietary fat should be 15-25% of total calories.

-Limit red meat. Eat more fish and poultry.

-Eliminate meat altogether - become vegetarian.

-Salty foods increase cancer risk.

-Herbs are great for seasoning foods.

-Tofu has lots of protein and is a great meat substitute.

-Squash has a lot of Vitamin A.

-Red peppers have a lot of Vitamins A & C.

-Shrimp is low in fat and high in protein.

-Onion can add lots of flavor without salt or fat.

-Broccoli is a great source of Vitamin C and fiber.

-Black cohosh relieves muscle spasms and reduces blood pressure.

-Licorice root reduces coughs and stabilizes blood sugar.

-Sarsaparilla root helps inflammation and fever.

-Blessed thistle helps inflammation, dysmenorrhea and allergies.

-Ginseng (Siberian) helps memory, fatigue, depression and stress.

-Sweating reduces the potassium level.

-Vitamin C helps hot flashes.

-Coffee increases the risk of bladder cancer 3-fold.

-Sugar contributes to thinning hair, tooth decay, fatigue and depression.

-Sugar decreases the T-cell immunity.

-One thousands teens die each year from cardiovascular attacks.

-Dairy foods contribute to mucus production.

-50% of the population is allergic to milk.

-Eating late doesn't allow the body to properly rest and repair.

-Diets low in fiber and water contribute to colon cancer.

-Obese parents have an 80% chance of having obese children.

-Green tea helps repair damaged tissue.

-Calcium causes the muscles to contract.

-Magnesium causes the muscles to relax.

-Magnesium helps relieve fatigue, constipation and migraines.

REFERENCES YOU MAY FIND HELPFUL

1. Atkins, Robert C., M.D., "Dr. Atkins' New Diet Revolution - The Amazing No-Hunger Weight-Loss Plan That Has Helped Millions Lose Weight and Keep It Off" Avon books, New York, NY, 1997.

2. Balch, James F., M.D., Phyllis A. Balch, CNC, "Prescriptions For Nutritional Healing", Avery Publishing Group, Garden City Park, NY, 1997.

3. Baldinger, Kathleen O'Bannon, "The World's Oldest Health Plan. Health, Nutrition and Healing From the Bible", Starburst, Lancaster, PA, 1994

4. Brenness, Lesley, "The Complete Book of Herbs. A Practical Guide to Growing and Using Herbs", Viking-Penguin, Inc., 1988.

5. Casper, Jean, "Miracle Cures: Dramatic New Scientific Discoveries Revealing the Healing Powers of Herbs, Vitamins and

Other Natural Remedies", Harper Collins Publishers, Inc., New York, NY, 1997.

6.   Courtis, Susan and Ramy Fraser, "Natural Healing For Women: Caring For Yourself With Herbs, Homeopathy and Essential Oils", Pandora Hammersmith, London, 1991.

7.   D'Adamo, Peter J., "Eat Right 4 Your Type", G.P. Putnam and Son, New York, 1996.

8.   Derfler, Astrid, "How to Grow Healing Herbs", Globe Communications Corporation, Boca Raton, FL, 1998.

9.   Diamond, Marilyn, Donald Burton Schnell, M.D., "Fitonics For Life - High Energy Lifestyle for the 21st Century", Avon Books, New York, NY, 1996.

10. Eades, Michael R., M.D. & Mary Dan Eades, M.D., "Protein Power: The High Protein/Low Carbohydrate Way to Lose Weight, Feel Fit and Boost Your Health In

Just Weeks!", Bantam Books, New York, NY, 1991.

11. Edmonds, John, "Foods That Melt Body Fat", Globe Communications Corporation, Boca Raton, FL, 1997.

12. Holy Bible, King James Version, Thomas Nelson Publishers, Nashville, TN, 1982.

13. Jakes, T.D., "Lay Aside The Weight - Take Control Of It Before It Takes Control Of You", Albury Publishing, Tulsa, OK, 1997.

14. James, Kathryn, "Burn Off Fat Forever - All Natural Wonder Foods", Micro May's, Lantona, FL, 1998.

15. Justice, L.A., "Shrink Your Tummy - A Fast Easy Weight Loss Plan", Globe Communications, Boca Raton, FL, 1997.

16. Katzenstern, Larry, "Secrets Of St. John's Wort", St. Martin Press, New York, NY, 1998.

17. Mandells, Earl R., Ph, PhD., "Food As Medicine: What You Can Eat To help Prevent Everything From Colds to Heart Disease To Cancer", Simon and Schuster, New York, NY, 1994.

18. Ody, Penelope, "Complete Medicinal Herbal", Doling Kindesley.

19. Richard, David, "Anoint Yourself With Oil For Radiant Health", Vital Health Publishing, Bloomington, IL, 1997.

20. Royal, Penny C., "Herbally Yours", Sound Nutrition, Payson, UT, 1985.

21. Sears, Barry, PhD, "Mastering The Zone: The Next Step In Achieving Super Health and Permanent Fat Loss", Harper Collins Publications, Inc., New York, NY, 1997.

22. Shamplina, Gwen, "The Weigh-Down Diet: Inspirational Way To Lose Weight, Stay Slim and Find A New You", Doubleday, New York, NY, 1997.

23.   Sheats, Cliff, "Lean Bodies - The Revolutionary New Approach To Losing Body Fat By Increasing Calories", The Summit Group, Fort Worth, TX, 1993.

24.   Wills, Judith, "Take Off 10 Years In 10 Weeks - A Change Your Life Program For The Outer You, The Vital You and The Inner You", Reader's Digest Association, Inc., Pleasantville, NY, 1997.

Permission was granted to use the breast and testicular exam diagrams found in Chapter 10 by Health Promotions Now, 215 Executive Dr. Moorestown, NJ 08057

HEALTH, WELLNESS & RESTORATION

The Complete Guide For Restoring
Your Health The Natural Way

It's What We've All Been Looking For

To order additional copies of this book, please send $23.60 (check or money order) plus $3.00 shipping and handling to:

> Denise Davis, M.D.
> P.O. Box 43264
> Cincinnati, Ohio 45243-0264

Ohio resident please add $1.40 sales tax for each book ordered.

To contact Dr. Denise Davis for lectures or workshops, please write to the above address.